DR. NOW'S
1200-Calorie Diet Plan

Dr. Nowzaradan's Balanced Meal Plan, Expert Tips, 365 Easy Recipes, and a Proven Formula for Rapid Weight Loss and Lasting Health.

JEFFREY M. JONES

COPYRIGHT ©

JEFFREY M. JONES

All rights reserved. No part of this book may be reproduced, stored in a retrieval system, or transmitted in any form or by any means, electronic, mechanical, Photocopying, recording, or otherwise, without the Prior written permission of the copyright holder, except In the case of brief quotations used in critical reviews or article.

DISCLAIMER

Please note the information contain within this document is for educational and entertainment purpose only. All effort has been executed to present accurate, up to date, reliable, and complete information. No warranties of any kind are declared or implied. Readers acknowledge that the author is not engaged in the rendering of legal, financial, medical or professional advice. The content within this book has been derived from various sources. Please consult a licensed professional before attempting any techniques outlined in this book. By reading this document the reader agrees that under no circumstances is the author responsible for any losses, direct or indirect, that are incurred as a result of the use of the information contained within this document, including, but not limited to, errors, omissions, or inaccuracies.

CONTENTS

INTRODUCTION 9

Understand the philosophy 10

Understanding the 1200 Calorie Diet 11

The Science behind the 1,200-Calorie Diet 12

Advantages of Low-Calorie Eating 13

Meal Preparation Tips: A Guide to Efficient and Healthy Eating. 14

Setting goals and expectations for your fitness journey. 15

Shopping Guide for Budget-Friendly Ingredients 17

CHAPTER ONE

BREAKFAST RECIPES

Greek Yogurt Parfait with Berries 19

Banana-Oat Pancakes. 20

Spinach and mushroom egg muffins. 21

Avocado Toast with Poached Egg 22

Almond Butter and Apple Smoothie. 23

CHAPTER TWO

LUNCH RECIPES 24

Grilled chicken salad with lemon dressing. 25

Zucchini Noodles with Marinara Sauce 26

Tuna lettuce wraps. 27

Lentil & Vegetable Soup 28

Turkey and Avocado Sandwich with Whole Grain 29

CHAPTER THREE

DINNER RECIPES 30

Baked salmon and asparagus 31

Grilled shrimp tacos with salsa. 32

Chicken stir-fry with brown rice 33

Turkey Meatballs with Zoodles 34

Stuffed bell peppers with quinoa 35

CHAPTER FOUR

SNACKS RECIPES 36

Veggie Sticks and Hummus 37

Roasted chickpeas 39

Cottage Cheese with Pineapple 40

Apple slices with cinnamon 41

Mixed nuts and seeds 42

CHAPTER FIVE

DESSERT RECIPES 43

Dark chocolate-dipped strawberries. 44

Chia pudding with almond milk 45

Baked Pears with Cinnamon 46

Protein-Rich Peanut Butter Cookies 47

Frozen Yogurt Bark and Fruit 49

BONUS RECIPES

Sweet Potato Breakfast Bowl. 50

Tomato and Spinach Omelet 51

Quinoa and Black Bean Bowl 52

Cod and Garlic Green Beans 54

Cauliflower Fried Rice 56

Greek yogurt with cucumber and dill is a refreshing and healthy snack. 57

Avocado-stuffed cherry tomatoes 58

Raspberry Coconut Energy Balls. 59

Banana Nice Cream. 60

Creating a Weekly Menu: A Strategic Approach 61

Prepping for Success: A Guide to Meal Planning and Preparation 64

60-Day Meal Plan 68

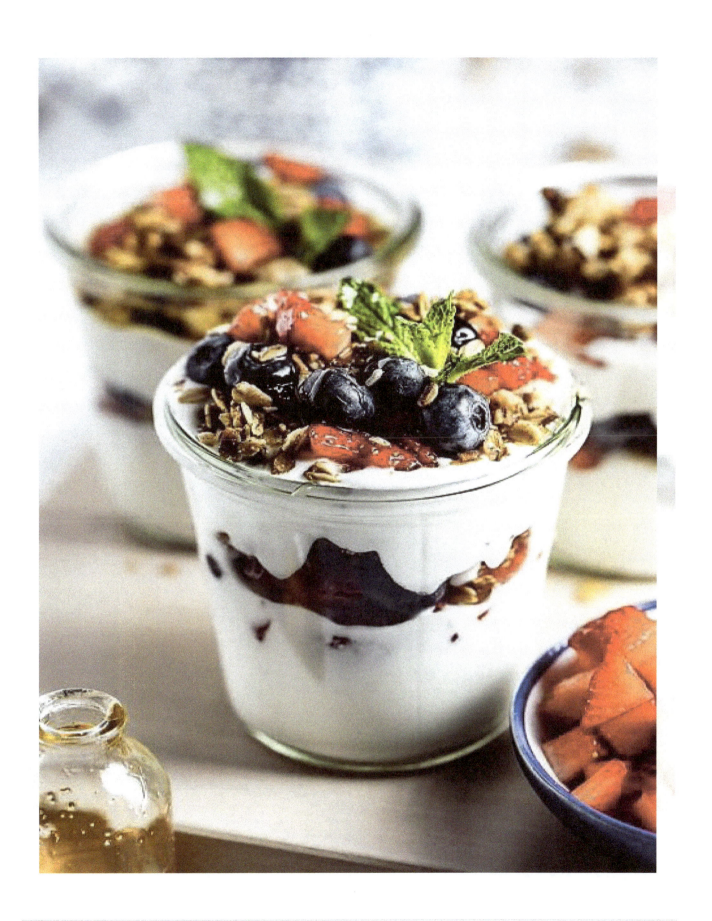

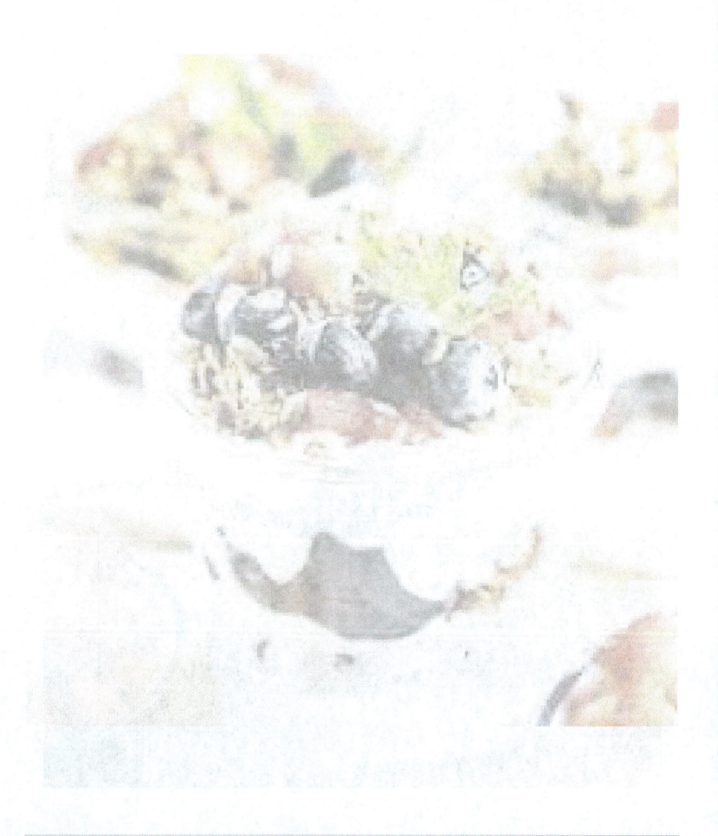

INTRODUCTION

Achieving and maintaining a healthy weight might seem like a daunting task, but with the appropriate direction and resources, you can transform your health objectives into long-term success. This book is inspired by Dr. Nowzaradan's well-known expertise in weight reduction and nutrition, and it provides a complete, science-backed strategy for losing weight and promoting long-term health.

Inside, you'll find a wealth of materials designed to make your weight reduction journey easier, more fun, and sustainable. From Dr. Now's tried-and-true balanced meal formula to 365 simple, economical, and tasty recipes, this book gives you the structure and diversity you need to stay motivated and fulfilled. Whether you want to lose weight, manage chronic diseases, or live a better lifestyle, these recipes and meal plans are designed to work effortlessly into your daily routine.

More than just diet, this book is about living better. Along with a 60-day food plan to get you started, you'll receive professional guidance, practical recommendations, and tactics for overcoming challenges. Dr. Now's method stresses balance, simplicity, and realistic goals, giving you the tools you need to achieve long-term outcomes.

Prepare to revolutionize your relationship with food, rediscover the joy of eating, and become a healthier, happier version of yourself. This is more than simply a diet; it's a long-term plan for a healthier life. Welcome to the beginning of your new journey!

Understand the philosophy

At the centre of this book is a straightforward yet transformational philosophy: Sustainable health begins with balance, simplicity, and consistency. Dr. Nowzaradan's approach does not involve crash diets, harsh limitations, or temporary remedies. Instead, it focuses on developing a happy relationship with food, supported by conscious decisions and lifelong techniques.

Dr. Now's balanced meal formula is based on nutrition research, emphasizing the value of nutrient-dense, whole meals while avoiding extra calories and unhealthy behaviours. This ideology promotes nourishing the body, aiding metabolism, and promoting general health while retaining the enjoyment of eating.

Key Tenets of Philosophy

- **Setting realistic goals leads to long-term success.**
  Quick results do not measure progress; rather, persistence and dedication do. Dr. Now stresses setting attainable goals and appreciating little accomplishments to preserve motivation and long-term success.
- **Nutrition is the foundation of health.**
  Weight reduction is more than just a matter of calorie intake and expenditure. It's about giving the body the nourishment it requires to flourish. This diet emphasizes lean proteins, healthy fats, and nutrient-dense veggies to feed the body and promote optimal performance.
- **Small changes lead to big results.**
  Adopting tiny, sustainable adjustments that fit into your daily life leads to long-term transformation. These practices eventually lead to a healthy lifestyle that feels natural and satisfying.
- **Flexibility Enables Progress**
  Life is unpredictable, as is the quest for greater health. By embracing flexibility—through food alternatives, replacements, and individualized strategies—you may adjust to problems without losing sight of your goals.
- **Healthy living should be affordable and accessible.**
  Eating healthy and caring for your body should not be considered a luxury. This attitude is grounded in realism, providing solutions that are appropriate for a variety of budgets, schedules, and tastes.

This book is about more than simply weight reduction; it is about developing a lifestyle that promotes both physical and mental health. It's about developing a long-term, pleasurable, and balanced attitude toward health that allows you to flourish rather than simply survive.

Understanding the 1200 Calorie Diet

What is a 1200-calorie diet?

A 1200-calorie diet is a very rigorous eating plan that restricts daily calorie consumption to 1200. This diet is frequently used for quick weight reduction or as a preoperative diet.

Who Should Consider a 1200 Calorie Diet?

A 1200-calorie diet should only be explored with the advice of a healthcare expert, such as a doctor or qualified dietitian. It may not be suitable for everyone or those with certain medical conditions.

Potential Benefits of a 1200 Calorie Diet

- **Fast weight reduction:** Significantly lowering calorie consumption might result in fast weight reduction in the near term.
- **Improved health markers:** In some situations, it may help with blood pressure, cholesterol, and blood sugar management.

Potential risks and side effects

The 1200-calorie diet may result in malnutrition, muscle loss, fatigue, and digestive issues.

- **Nutrient Deficiencies:** Inadequate intake of vital vitamins and minerals can have a detrimental influence on overall health.
- **Yo-Yo Dieting:** Rapid weight reduction frequently results in weight return, particularly if the diet is not sustainable.

Important Considerations

- **Speak a Healthcare Professional**: Before beginning any restricted diet, speak with a healthcare practitioner to confirm it is safe and appropriate for your specific requirements.
- **Prioritize Nutrient-Dense Foods:** Include fruits, vegetables, lean proteins, and whole grains in your diet.
- **Stay Hydrated:** Drink plenty of water throughout the day.
- **Listen to Your Body:** Pay attention to hunger and fullness cues. Avoid extreme restrictions. A balanced and sustained strategy for weight loss is usually more effective in the long run.

It's important to realize that a 1200-calorie diet isn't a long-term weight-management strategy. It is critical to have a long-term strategy that promotes your entire health and well-being.

Do you want to learn more about a certain component of the 1200-calorie diet, such as its hazards, advantages, or how to develop a balanced meal plan?

The Science behind the 1,200-Calorie Diet

The 1200-calorie diet is based on the fundamental premise of weight loss: calorie deficit. When you consume fewer calories than you burn, your body uses up its energy reserves, resulting in weight loss.

Here's a breakdown of the science:

- **Caloric Deficit Energy Balance**: Our bodies balance calorie intake and expenditure.
- **Weight loss:** When we eat fewer calories than we spend, we generate a calorie deficit, forcing the body to use stored energy, mostly fat.

Metabolic Adaptation

- **Metabolic Slowdown:** As calorie intake decreases, your body may slow metabolism to preserve energy. This might make losing weight more difficult over time.
- **How to Counteract Metabolic Slowdown:** To fight this, eat a well-balanced diet and exercise often.

Macronutrient Balance.

While calorie restriction is critical, it's also necessary to maintain a balanced macronutrient intake. Protein is necessary for muscle preservation and repair.

- Carbohydrates fuel the body and brain.
- Fats aid hormone synthesis and nutrition absorption.

Potential risk and considerations:

While a 1200-calorie diet can be successful for weight reduction, it's vital to be aware of the following risks:

- **Malnutrition:** If not properly designed, restrictive diets might result in dietary shortages.
- **Muscle Loss:** Excessive calorie restriction might result in muscle loss, which slows metabolism.
- **Yo-Yo Dieting:** Rapid weight reduction frequently results in weight return, particularly if the diet is not sustainable.

To reduce these hazards, it's important to:

- **Prioritize Nutrient-Dense Foods:** Focus on consuming whole foods like fruits, vegetables, lean proteins, and whole grains.
- **Stay Hydrated:** Drink plenty of water throughout the day.
- **Listen to Your Body:** Pay attention to hunger and fullness cues.
- **Avoid Extreme Restrictions:** A balanced and sustainable approach to weight loss.

Understanding the science behind the 1200-calorie diet and following the required precautions allows you to utilize it as a tool to attain your weight reduction objectives in a safe and effective manner.

Advantages of Low-Calorie Eating

A low-calorie diet, when followed appropriately, can provide a variety of health benefits. Here are some of the main advantages:

Weight Management

- **Weight Loss:** Consuming fewer calories than you expend is a key factor for weight loss.
- **Reduced Body Fat:** A calorie deficit promotes the body to burn stored fat for energy.
- **Improved body composition:** A well-balanced, low-calorie diet can help you maintain or gain muscle mass while losing body fat.
- A low-calorie diet can lower high blood pressure and minimize the risk of heart disease by decreasing cholesterol and inflammation.
- A low-calorie diet helps improve blood sugar control, particularly for those with diabetes or prediabetes.
- Additionally, it can lower the risk of some cancers. Some studies indicate that a calorie-restricted diet may lower the risk of some forms of cancer.

Improved Well-Being

- **Increased Energy Levels:** A low-calorie diet can give long-lasting energy.
- **Improved Mood:** A nutritious diet may have a favorable influence on both mental health and mood.
- A well-balanced diet can improve sleep quality, while nutrient-rich, low-calorie meals can enhance cognitive performance.

Important Considerations

- **Speak to a healthcare professional:** Before beginning a new diet, speak with a healthcare practitioner to confirm it is safe and appropriate for your specific circumstances.
- **Balanced Nutrition:** A low-calorie diet should be well-balanced, with plenty of nutrient-dense foods including fruits, vegetables, lean meats, and whole grains.
- **Hydration:** Drink lots of water throughout the day to keep hydrated and promote good health.
- Pay attention to your body's hunger and fullness cues. Avoid extreme restrictions for long-term weight reduction success.

Following a well-planned low-calorie diet will help you lose weight, improve your general health, and increase your quality of life.

Meal Preparation Tips: A Guide to Efficient and Healthy Eating.

Meal planning is an excellent method to save time, decrease stress, and eat better. Here are some suggestions to help you get started:

Planning is key.

- **Make a Weekly Meal Plan:** Plan your weekly meals around your schedule and dietary requirements.
- **Make a Grocery List:** To minimize impulse purchases, develop a comprehensive grocery list based on your meal plan.

Efficient preparation techniques.

- Wash and chop produce ahead of time and store in airtight containers.
- Cook grains in bulk and store them in the refrigerator or freezer.
- Marinate proteins to tenderize and add flavor.
- Prepare sauces and dressings ahead of time and store in jars or bottles.

Smart Storage Solutions.

- Use airtight containers to keep food fresh and prevent spoilage.
- Freeze cooked meals, soups, sauces, and stocks for later use.
- Organize your fridge to easily find ingredients and reduce food waste.

Quick and Easy Meal Ideas

- **Salad Bowls:** Make a quick and healthy dinner using pre-cooked grains, roasted veggies, and protein sources.
- **Sandwich and Wrap Combos:** Use a range of ingredients, including roasted chicken, grilled vegetables, or hummus, to make various sandwiches and wraps.
- **Pasta Salads:** Toss cooked pasta with veggies, protein, and a delicious dressing.
- **Soup and Stew:** Make big amounts of soup or stew and freeze them for later.

Additional Tips

- Involve your family in meal planning and preparation.
- Be flexible and adjust your plan as needed.
- Experiment with new recipes and ingredients to keep things interesting.
- Don't be afraid to ask for help.

- If you are feeling overwhelmed, contact a friend or family member for assistance with meal preparation.

By following these suggestions, you may simplify your meal prep process, save time, and eat healthier, more flavorful meals.

Setting goals and expectations for your fitness journey.

Understanding your "why"

Before beginning a workout practice, it is critical to understand your reasons. Why do you want to get fit? Is it to enhance health, lose weight, gain vitality, or boost self-esteem? Having a clear "why" can help you stay motivated, especially in difficult situations.

Setting SMART goals

Once you've determined your "why," define clear, measurable, attainable, relevant, and time-bound (SMART) objectives. Here's an example.

To achieve my goal of losing 10 pounds, I will check my weight weekly, progressively increase my activity intensity, and cut my calorie consumption.

- **Relevant:** Losing weight will boost my health and self-confidence.
- **Time-bound:** I plan to attain my objective within 3 months.

Realistic Expectations

- **Progress Takes Time:** Remember that major changes take time. Be patient with yourself and appreciate tiny achievements.
- **Listen to Your Body:** Avoid pushing yourself too hard. Rest when necessary and prevent overtraining.
- **Embrace Setbacks:** Everyone has setbacks. Learn from them and turn them into chances for growth.

Create a supportive environment.

- **Find an exercise buddy:** An exercise companion helps keep you motivated and accountable.
- **Join a Fitness Community:** Meet like-minded people who share your fitness goals.
- **Seek professional guidance:** For tailored guidance, see a fitness trainer or licensed nutritionist.

Setting clear objectives, controlling expectations, and establishing a supportive atmosphere will help you launch on a successful fitness journey.

Essential Kitchen Tools

A well-stocked kitchen is essential for successful meal preparation and cooking. Here are some basic tools to help you get started:

- **Knives:** A good pair of knives is a need. A chef's knife, a serrated knife, and a paring knife are necessary.
- **Cutting Board**: A robust cutting board protects counters and provides a firm platform for chopping.
- **Pots and Pans:** Having a selection of pots and pans in different sizes is vital for preparing various foods.
- **Cookware:** A high-quality skillet, saucepan, and stockpot are required.
  Baking Sheets: These flexible sheets may be used for baking, roasting, and broiling.
- **Mixing Bowls:** Having a variety of mixing bowls of different sizes is handy for creating recipes.
- **Measuring Cups and Spoons:** Accurate measurements are crucial for baking and cooking.
- **Whisk:** A whisk is essential for whisking eggs, sauces, and batters.
- **Spatulas**: Spatulas are used for flipping, scraping, and spreading.
- **Tongs:** Tongs are helpful for flipping and turning food without piercing it.

Shopping Guide for Budget-Friendly Ingredients

Here are some suggestions for buying on a budget:

To minimize impulsive purchases, plan your meals and make a shopping list. Stick to the list to avoid buying unneeded things.
To save money, consider buying non-perishable things like rice, pasta, and canned goods in bulk. Generic brands can provide comparable quality at a reduced price. Seasonal produce is frequently cheaper and fresher.

- **Use Coupons and Discounts:** Take advantage of coupons, discounts, and loyalty programs.
- **Cook at Home:** Cooking at home is often cheaper than dining out.
- **Pack Your Lunch:** Packing your lunch may save you money and promote healthy eating habits.
- **Freeze Leftovers:** Freezing leftovers can reduce food waste and save money.

By following these guidelines, you may equip your kitchen and supply it with low-cost ingredients. Happy cooking!

CHAPTER ONE

BREAKFAST

RECIPES

Breakfast is an essential part of the 1200-calorie diet, providing the necessary energy to start the day while keeping you satisfied. These recipes are designed to be both nutritious and fulfilling, offering a mix of protein, fiber, and healthy fats. Whether you're in the mood for something sweet, savory, or quick and easy, these breakfast ideas are tailored to fit within your calorie goals while fuelling your body for the day ahead. Enjoy tasty, balanced meals that set a positive tone for the rest of your day!

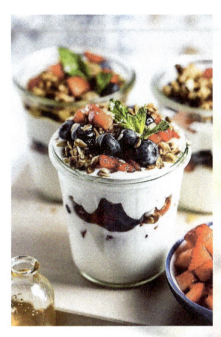

Greek Yogurt Parfait with Berries

Prep Time: 5 minutes

Total Time: 5 minutes.

Ingredients:

- 1 cup plain Greek yogurt.
- 1/2 cup mixed berries.
- Add 1 tablespoon of honey (optional) and 2 tablespoons of granola.

Directions:

- In a glass, combine Greek yogurt and berries, sprinkle with honey, and top with granola. Serve immediately or refrigerate till later.

Nutrition (Per Serving):

- Calories: 180, Protein: 12 grams, Carbohydrate: 24 g, Fat: 3g

Health Benefits:

- High in protein, probiotics for intestinal health, antioxidants from berries, and fiber.

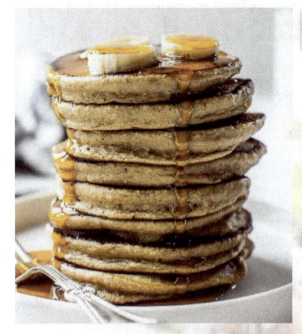

Banana-Oat Pancakes.

Prep Time: 5 minutes

Cooking Time: 10 minutes.

Total time: 15 minutes.

Ingredients:

- Two ripe bananas.
- 1 cup rolled oats and 2 eggs.
- One teaspoon of baking powder.
- 1/2 teaspoon cinnamon (optional)
- One teaspoon of vanilla extract (optional)
- One pinch of salt.
- To fry, use cooking spray or a little coconut oil.

Directions:
1. In a blender or food processor, combine the oats until they have a flour-like consistency.
2. Combine the bananas, eggs, baking powder, cinnamon, vanilla, and salt with the oats and mix until smooth.
3. Heat a nonstick pan or griddle over medium heat, then gently coat with cooking spray or coconut oil.
4. Pour tiny amounts of batter into the skillet and cook for 2–3 minutes per side until golden brown.
5. If wanted, serve warm with honey or fresh fruit drizzle.

Nutritional information (per serving): Calorie: 250, Protein: 9 grams, Carbohydrate: 35g, Fat: 8g , Fiber: 4 grams, Sugar: 12 grams.

Health Benefits:

High in Fiber: Oats and bananas contain fiber, which promotes digestive health and helps you feel fuller for longer.
Good Source of Potassium: Bananas are high in potassium, which is vital for heart health and muscular function.
Protein-Rich: Eggs provide protein for muscle upkeep and repair.
Natural Sweetness: Bananas serve as a natural sweetener, minimizing the need for additional sugar.

This recipe makes around 3 to 4 pancakes per serving, making it ideal for a healthy breakfast for one person. For a balanced meal, serve with a protein-rich side dish or a healthy fat source like almond butter or avocado.

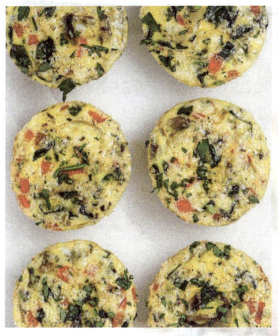

Spinach and mushroom egg muffins.

Prep time: 10 minutes

Cooking time: 15-20 minutes.

Total time: 25-30 minutes.

Ingredients:

- Six big eggs.
- 1 cup freshly chopped spinach.
- ½ cup chopped mushrooms.
- 1/4 cup of low-fat cheese (optional).
- Add salt and pepper to taste.
- Using cooking spray or olive oil to grease

Directions:
1. Heat the oven to 375°F (190°C) and butter a muffin pan.
2. Sauté the mushrooms and spinach until they soften.
3. Whisk the eggs with the salt and pepper, and then add the cooked veggies.
4. Transfer the egg mixture to the muffin tray.
5. Bake the eggs for 15-20 minutes, or until completely set.

Nutritional information (Per muffin): Calories: 80, Protein: 7 grams, Carbs: 2 grams, Fat: 5g, Fiber: 1 g.

Health Benefits:

- **High Protein:** Eggs promote muscle development and repair.
- **Rich in Vitamins:** Spinach contains iron, calcium, and antioxidants.
- **Low in Carbs:** Excellent choice for a low-carbohydrate diet.
- **Good for Digestion:** Spinach and mushrooms are high in fiber, which promotes digestive health.

Portion per Day: A normal serving size is 2-3 muffins, making it a substantial breakfast or snack. For added energy, pair with a side of fruit or a small serving of nutritious grains.

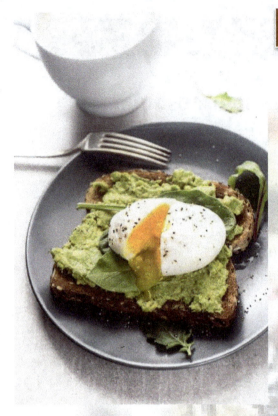

Avocado Toast with Poached Egg

Preparation Time: 5 minutes

Cooking Time: 5 minutes

Total time: 10 minutes.

Ingredients:

- One ripe avocado.
- 1 slices of whole-grain bread and 1 big egg.
- Season to taste with salt and pepper, and optionally add red pepper flakes or lemon juice.

Directions:

1. Toast bread till desired level.
2. Mash the avocado with salt, pepper, and any other ingredients.
3. Cook the egg in boiling water for 3–4 minutes.
4. Spread mashed avocado over the bread, then top with a poached egg and serve.

Health Benefits

- **Rich in Healthy Fats**: Avocado provides monounsaturated fats, which support heart health, reduce bad cholesterol, and improve overall cardiovascular function.
- **High-Quality Protein**: The poached egg is an excellent source of protein, aiding in muscle repair and maintaining a feeling of fullness.
- **Packed with Fiber**: Whole-grain toast and avocado contribute dietary fiber, promoting good digestion and stabilizing blood sugar levels.
- **Nutrient-Dense**: This meal offers vitamins like B6, E, and K (from avocado) and essential minerals like potassium and magnesium, which help regulate blood pressure.
- **Low in Calories**: It's a nutrient-packed, low-calorie option, perfect for weight management and sustaining energy throughout the day.

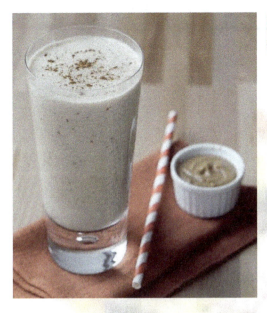

Almond Butter and Apple Smoothie.

Prep Time: 5 minutes

Total Time: 5 minutes.

Ingredients:

- 1 medium apple, chopped
- 1 tablespoon almond butter, 1/2 cup almond milk.
- 1/2 cup Greek yogurt.
- One teaspoon honey (optional)

Directions:

1. Blend all ingredients until smooth.
2. Pour into a glass and serve immediately.

Health Benefits:

Both recipes contain healthy fats, fiber, and protein. Avocado toast delivers heart-healthy lipids, but an almond butter and apple smoothie has antioxidants and energy-boosting minerals.

CHAPTER TWO

LUNCH

RECIPES

Lunch is an essential part of your daily meals, offering the perfect opportunity to refuel and recharge for the rest of the day. These lunch recipes are designed to be both nutritious and satisfying while fitting into your 1200-calorie plan. Whether you're looking for a quick bite or a more filling dish, these recipes incorporate a variety of wholesome ingredients—lean proteins, healthy fats, and fiber-rich vegetables—to keep you energized and on track with your goals. Enjoy a delicious, balanced meal that fuels your body and keeps you feeling satisfied.

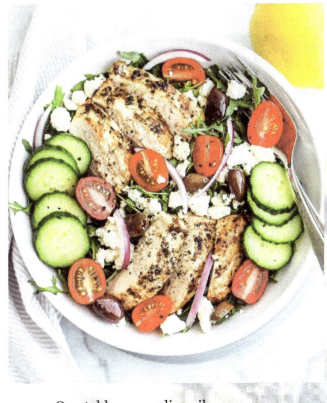

Grilled chicken salad with lemon dressing.

Prep Time: 10 minutes

Cooking Time: 10 minutes.

Total time: 20 minutes.

Ingredients:

- 1 boneless, skinless chicken breast, 4 cups mixed greens (spinach, arugula, and lettuce),
- ½ sliced cucumber, and 1 cup halved cherry tomatoes.
- One tablespoon olive oil.
- Season with salt and pepper to taste.
- Add 1 tablespoon fresh lemon juice.
- One teaspoon Dijon mustard (optional)

Directions:

1. Season chicken breast with salt, pepper, and olive oil. Grill for 6-7 minutes per side until thoroughly done.
2. Combine the greens, cucumbers, and tomatoes in a dish.
3. Slice the chicken and arrange on top of the salad.
4. Combine the lemon juice and Dijon mustard, and then sprinkle it over the salad.

Health Benefits:

- **Lean Protein**: Chicken is abundant in protein, which helps maintain and rebuild muscles.
- **Antioxidants:** Fresh veggies provide vitamins and antioxidants.
- **Healthy Fats:** Olive oil contains healthy fats, which promote heart health.

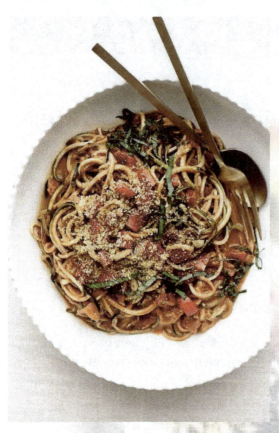

Zucchini Noodles with Marinara Sauce

Prep Time: 10 minutes

Cooking Time: 5 minutes.

Total time: 15 minutes.

Ingredients:

- 2 spiralized medium zucchinis and 1 cup marinara sauce.
- 1 tsp. olive oil. Season with salt and pepper.
- Optional: fresh basil

Directions:

1. Saute zucchini noodles in olive oil for 3–4 minutes.
2. Heat the marinara sauce in a separate pan.
3. Serve zucchini noodles with sauce and fresh basil.

Health Benefits:

- Zucchini has low calories, high fiber, and vitamins.

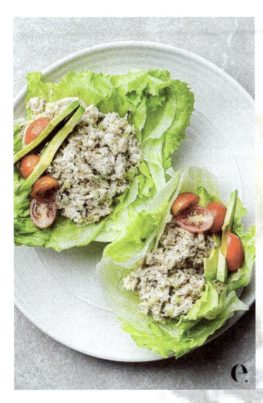

Tuna lettuce wraps.

Prep Time: 5 minutes.

Cooking Time: None.

Total Time: 5 minutes.

Ingredients:

- 1 can drain tuna and 2 tbsp. Greek yogurt.
- 1 teaspoon mustard, 4 big lettuce leaves, salt, and pepper to taste.

Directions:

1. Combine tuna, Greek yogurt, mustard, salt, and pepper.
2. Spoon the mixture into lettuce leaves and wrap.

Health Benefits:

- High in protein, low in carbohydrates, and high in omega-3 fatty acids.

Lentil & Vegetable Soup

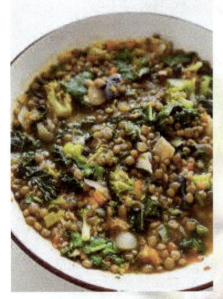

Prep Time: 10 minutes

Cooking Time: 30 minutes.

Total time: 40 minutes.

Ingredients:

- One cup of dried lentils.
- One chopped carrot
- 1 celery stem, chopped
- 1 onion, chopped
- 2 garlic cloves, minced
- 4 cups vegetable broth and 1 can chop tomatoes.
- 1 teaspoon of cumin.
- Add salt and pepper to taste.

Directions:
1. In a large saucepan, cook the onion, carrot, celery, and garlic in a little olive oil until softened.
2. Combine the vegetable broth, diced tomatoes, lentils, cumin, salt, and pepper in the saucepan.
3. Bring to a boil, then decrease the heat and simmer for 25–30 minutes or until the lentils are cooked.
4. Adjust the spice as needed and serve hot.

Nutritional information (per serving): Calories: 180, Protein: 12 grams, Carbohydrate: 32g, Fat: 1g, Fiber: 14 grams, Sugar: 6 grams.

Health Benefits:

- **High in Protein:** Lentils provide plant-based protein, which is crucial for muscle repair and growth.
- **High in Fiber:** Lentils and vegetables include fiber, which promotes digestive health and helps to maintain healthy blood sugar levels.
- **Low in Fat:** This soup is low in fat, which is good for your heart.
- **Packed with Nutrients:** Vegetables and legumes include a variety of vitamins, including folate, potassium, and iron.

Portion per Day: This soup is filling and suitable for lunch or dinner. A normal serving size is 1-1.5 cups, which is suitable for a balanced, calorie-conscious diet.

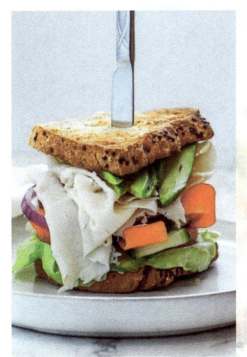

Turkey and Avocado Sandwich with Whole Grain

Prep Time: 5 minutes.

Cooking Time: None.

Total Time: 5 minutes.

Ingredients:

- 2 pieces of whole grain bread; 3 ounces sliced turkey breast.
- 1/2 avocado, sliced
- Leafy greens (spinach, lettuce)
- Mustard or Hummus (optional)

Directions:

1. Toast or use fresh bread.
2. Arrange the pieces of turkey on one slice of bread.
3. Add avocado and leafy leaves.
4. Spread mustard or hummus on the second slice of bread, then seal the sandwich.
5. Slice and serve.

Nutritional information (per serving): Calories: 350, Protein: 30 grams, Carbohydrate: 32g, Fat: 15g, Fiber: 9 grams, Sugar: 5 grams.

Health Benefits:

- **High in Protein**: Turkey contains lean protein, which promotes muscular growth and keeps you fuller for longer.
- **High in Healthy Fats**: Avocados include monounsaturated fats, which promote heart health and lower inflammation.
- **High in Fiber:** Whole grain bread and avocado increase daily fiber consumption, which promotes digestive health and satiety.
- **Nutrition Dense:** Packed with vital vitamins and minerals, such as potassium and folate.

Portion per Day: This sandwich may be a satisfying lunch or dinner. One sandwich is usually plenty for most people, especially when served with a side salad or some veggie sticks.

CHAPTER THREE

DINNER

RECIPES

Dinner is an important meal to cap off your day, offering the opportunity to nourish your body with a variety of nutrient-dense ingredients. These dinner recipes are designed to be both satisfying and healthy, fitting seamlessly into your 1200-calorie plan. From lean proteins to vibrant vegetables, each dish balances flavor and nutrition, ensuring you enjoy a delicious and wholesome meal while keeping your calorie intake in check. Whether you're cooking for yourself or preparing a meal for the family, these recipes offer the perfect way to finish the day on a high note.

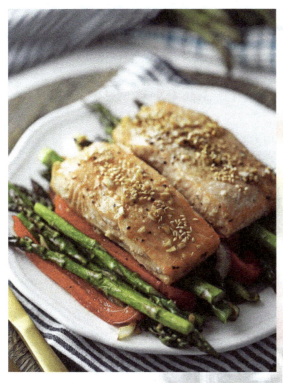

Baked salmon and asparagus

Prep Time: 10 minutes

Cooking Time: 15-20 minutes.

Total time: 25-30 minutes.

Ingredients:

- 2 salmon fillets, 1 bunch of asparagus,
- 1 tbsp olive oil, salt and pepper to taste, and optional lemon wedges.

Directions:
1. Preheat your oven to 400°F (200°C).
2. Arrange the salmon fillets and asparagus on a baking pan.
3. Drizzle with olive oil, then season with salt and pepper.
4. Bake for 15-20 minutes or until the salmon is well cooked and readily flaked.

Health Benefits:

- **Rich in Omega-3s:** Salmon contains heart-healthy lipids.
- **Rich in Protein:** Promotes muscle maintenance and restoration.
- **Fiber and Vitamins:** Asparagus contains fiber, folate, and vitamins A, C, and K.

Portion per Day: This recipe feeds two people and is ideal for a light yet hearty dinner. To add more greens, serve with a small side salad.

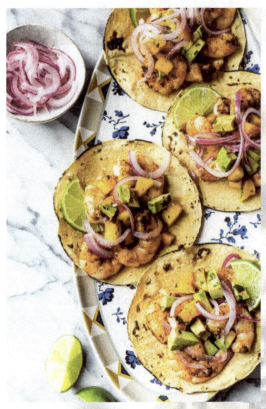

Grilled shrimp tacos with salsa.

Prep Time: 10 minutes

Cooking Time: 8-10 minutes.

Total time: 18-20 minutes.

Ingredients:

- 1 pound peeled and deveined shrimp; 1 tablespoon olive oil
- 1 teaspoon of cumin.
- One teaspoon of chili powder
- One lime, juiced
- Eight tiny corn tortillas
- Salsa with tomato, onion, cilantro, and lime.
- Fresh cilantro for garnish.

Directions:

1. Season shrimp with olive oil, cumin, chili powder, and lime juice.
2. Grill the shrimp for 2–3 minutes per side.
3. Warm tortillas before assembling tacos with shrimp and salsa.
4. Garnish with fresh cilantro.

Health Benefits:

Protein-Rich: Shrimp contains lean protein.
High in Vitamins: Salsa contains antioxidants like tomatoes and vitamins A and C.
Low-Carb: Excellent low-carb meal choice.

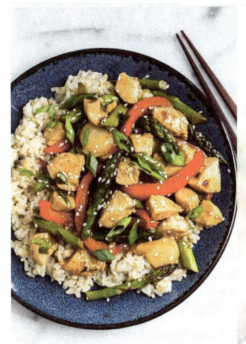

Chicken stir-fry with brown rice

Prep Time: 10 minutes

Cooking Time: 15-20 minutes

Total Time: 25-30 minutes.

Ingredients:

- 2 thinly sliced chicken breasts and 2 cups mixed veggies (e.g., bell peppers, carrots, and broccoli).
- 2 tablespoons soy sauce (low sodium) one tablespoon of olive oil.
- 1 teaspoon grated ginger and 1 cup cooked brown rice.

Directions:
1. Heat the olive oil in a skillet and cook the chicken until done.
2. Add the veggies and stir fry for 5–7 minutes.
3. Stir in the soy sauce and ginger, and simmer for an additional 2–3 minutes.
4. Serve with cooked brown rice.

Health Benefits:

- **Lean Protein:** Chicken contains low-fat protein.
- Brown rice and veggies are high in fiber, which aids digestion.
- **Packed with Vitamins:** Vegetables provide critical vitamins and minerals.

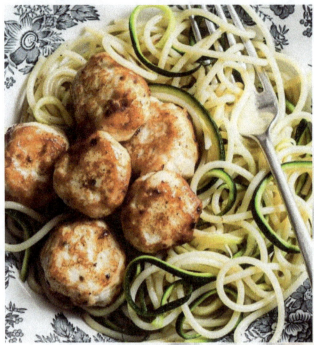

Turkey Meatballs with Zoodles

Prep Time: 15 minutes

Cooking Time: 20 minutes.

Total time: 35 minutes.

Ingredients:

- 1 pound ground turkey; 1/4 cup breadcrumbs (or almond flour for a low-carb alternative).
- 1 egg
- 1/4 cup grated parmesan cheese.
- 2 zucchini spiralized into noodles.
- One cup marinara sauce.
- Season with salt and pepper to taste. Add 1 tablespoon olive oil.

Directions:

1. Preheat your oven to 375°F (190°C).
2. Combine turkey, breadcrumbs, egg, Parmesan, salt, and pepper; shape into meatballs.
3. Bake the meatballs for 15 to 20 minutes.
4. Cook the zoodles in olive oil for 2-3 minutes, until soft.
5. Garnish zoodles with marinara sauce and meatballs.

Health Benefits:

- **High in Protein:** Turkey contains lean protein that promotes muscle regeneration.
- **Low-Carb:** Zoodles are a low-carb alternative to pasta that is high in fiber and vitamins.
- **Reduced-fat:** Using ground turkey keeps the meal reduced in fat while still providing a good source of nutrients.

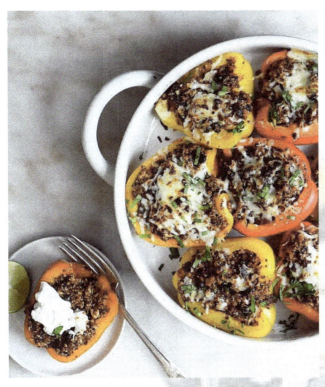

Stuffed bell peppers with quinoa

Prep Time: 15 minutes

Cooking Time: 30 minutes.

Total time: 45 minutes

Ingredients:

- Four bell peppers of any color.
- 1 cup cooked quinoa and 1 can drained and rinsed black beans.
- 1 cup corn kernels, fresh or frozen.
- 1 teaspoon cumin and 1 teaspoon chili powder.
- One tablespoon olive oil.
- Season with salt and pepper to taste.
- Optional: add 1/2 cup shredded cheese.

Directions:

1. Preheat the oven to 375°F (190°C).
2. Cut the tops of the bell peppers and remove the seeds.
3. In a bowl, add the quinoa, black beans, corn, cumin, chili powder, olive oil, salt, and pepper.
4. Fill the peppers with the mixture and set in a baking tray.
5. Sprinkle with cheese if desired, and bake for 25–30 minutes.

Health Benefits:

- **High in Protein and Fiber:** Quinoa and black beans include plant-based protein and fiber, which improve digestion and keep you satisfied.
- **Antioxidant-Rich:** Bell peppers are high in vitamins A and C, which benefit the immune system and the skin.
- **Low in Fat:** This meal is inherently low in fat, particularly with the optional cheese toppings.

CHAPTER FOUR

SNACKS

RECIPES

Snacking is an important part of maintaining energy levels throughout the day, but choosing healthy, nutrient-packed options is key. These snack recipes are designed to keep you on track with your 1200-calorie meal plan while satisfying cravings in a wholesome way. Whether you're looking for something sweet, savory, or a combination of both, these snacks offer the perfect balance of protein, fiber, and healthy fats. Enjoy a quick bite that will not only keep you satisfied but also nourish your body.

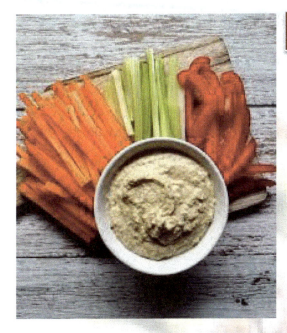

Veggie Sticks and Hummus

Preparation time: 15 minutes.

Ingredients:

For the Hummus:

- 1 cans (15 ounces) washed and drained chickpeas
- 1/4 cup tahini 1/4 cup fresh lemon juice
- 2 minced garlic cloves 1/4 teaspoon salt
- 1/4 teaspoon ground cumin 1/4 cup cold water

For the Veggie Sticks:

- To make the sticks, peel and chop 1 carrot, 1 cucumber, 1 red bell pepper, and 1 green bell pepper.

Directions

1. Prepare the hummus: In a food processor, mix the chickpeas, tahini, lemon juice, garlic, salt, and cumin.
Process until smooth, adding cold water gradually to get the desired consistency.
Taste and adjust spices as necessary.

2. Prepare the Veggie Sticks: Wash and chop the veggies into similar-sized sticks.

3. Serve: Place the hummus in a serving bowl. Place the vegetable sticks on a dish. Serve the hummus with the vegetable sticks for dipping.

Nutritional value (per serving): Calories range from 150 to 200, Protein: 5-8g, Fat: 5-10g, Carbohydrates: 15-20g, Fiber: 4-6 grams

Health benefits:

- **High in Fiber:** Vegetables and chickpeas contain fiber, which assists digestion and enhances fullness.
- **High in Protein:** Hummus contains a lot of plant-based protein, which is necessary for muscle repair and development.
- **Nutrient-Dense:** Vegetables include a range of vitamins, minerals, and antioxidants.

- **Heart-Healthy:** The unsaturated fats in hummus and fiber in veggies can help decrease cholesterol.
- **Hydrating:** Vegetables' high water content promotes hydration.

Portions per Day:

Consider this a snack or light meal. Portion size should be adjusted to meet your specific calorie requirements and dietary objectives.

Note: This is a generic recipe. Add other veggies, such as celery, broccoli, or jicama, to make it your own. You may also use other herbs and spices to flavor the hummus.

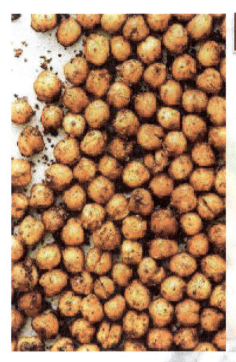

Roasted chickpeas

Prep Time: 15 minutes

Cooking Time: 30-40 minutes

Ingredients:

- 1 can (15 ounces) washed and drained chickpeas,
- 2 tablespoons olive oil,
- 1 teaspoon paprika,
- 1/2 teaspoon garlic powder,
- 1/4 teaspoon cayenne pepper and 1/4 teaspoon salt.

Directions:

1. Preheat your oven to 400°F (200°C).
2. Prepare chickpeas: Spread the chickpeas over a paper towel to dry completely.
3. Season Chickpeas: In a large bowl, toss chickpeas with olive oil, paprika, garlic powder, cayenne pepper, and salt. Toss to coat evenly.
4. Roast Chickpeas: Place the seasoned chickpeas in a single layer on a baking sheet lined with parchment paper.
5. Bake: Roast in a preheated oven for 30 to 40 minutes, until golden brown and crispy. Stir halfway through to ensure uniform browning.
6. Cool and Serve: Allow chickpeas to cool fully before serving. Keep in an airtight container at room temperature.

Nutritional value (per serving): Calories range from 150 to 200. Protein: 5-8g, Fat: 5-10g Carbohydrates: 15-20g, Fiber: 4-6 grams

Health benefits:

- **High in Protein:** A plant-based protein source.
- **Rich in Fiber:** Promotes digestion and satiety.
- **Nutrient-Dense:** Packed with vitamins, minerals, and antioxidants.
- **Heart-Healthy:** Low in saturated fat and high in fiber, which can help lower cholesterol.
- **Versatile Snack:** Can be eaten on their own or mixed into salads, soups, or yogurt.

Portions per Day: A half-cup portion can be a filling snack.

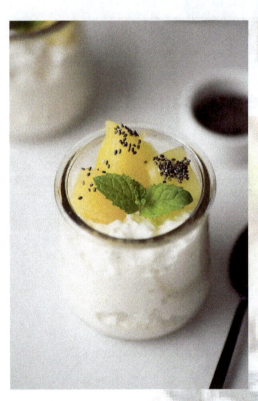

Cottage Cheese with Pineapple

Preparation time: 5 minutes.

Ingredients:

Ingredients:

- 1 cup cottage cheese,
- 1/2 cup diced fresh pineapple, a drizzle of honey, and a sprinkle of cinnamon (optional).

Directions;

1. Combine Ingredients: In a bowl, mix together cottage cheese and diced pineapple.
2. Sweeten (Optional): For added taste, use honey and cinnamon.
3. Serve immediately and enjoy.

Nutritional value (per serving): Calories: 150-200, Protein: 12-15 g, Fat: 5-8 g, Carbs: 10-15 g, Calcium: 20-25% of daily value.

Health benefits:

- High in protein for tissue repair.
- High in calcium for strong bones and teeth. Good source of vitamin C for immunity and iron absorption.
- Low in calories for weight management. A refreshing and satisfying snack.

Portions per Day: One-cup servings can be a filling snack or light breakfast.

Note: These nutritional values are approximate and may differ based on the brand and serving size. Always check the nutritional information on the product label.

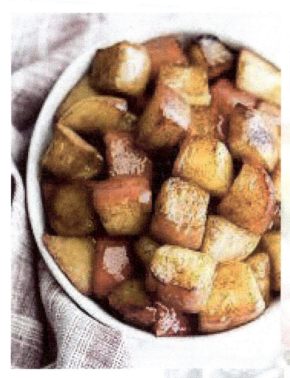

Apple slices with cinnamon

Preparation time: 5 minutes.

Ingredients:

- 1 big apple, cored and sliced
- 1/4 teaspoon ground cinnamon

Directions:

1. Slice Apple: Cut the apple into small pieces.
2. Add cinnamon: Sprinkle cinnamon on the apple slices.
3. Serve immediately and enjoy.

Nutritional value (per serving):

This food's nutritional value depends on apple size and cinnamon use. Apples, on the other hand, have high levels of fiber, vitamin C, and antioxidants. Cinnamon is anti-inflammatory and can help control blood sugar levels.

Health benefits:

- High fiber content promotes digestion and fullness.
- High vitamin C content boosts immunity and iron absorption.
- Antioxidant powerhouse protects cells from damage.
- Anti-inflammatory properties reduce inflammation.
- Blood sugar regulation helps stabilize levels.

Portions per Day: A medium-sized apple may make a tasty snack.

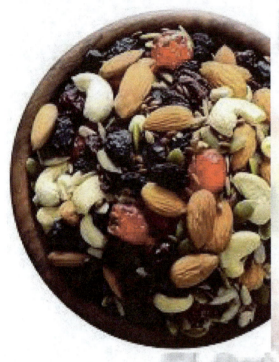

Mixed nuts and seeds

Preparation time: 5 minutes.

Ingredients:

- 1/4 cup almonds,
- 1/4 cup walnuts,
- 1/4 cup pumpkin seeds,
- 1/4 cup sunflower seeds,
- 1 tablespoon chia seeds, and
- 1 tablespoon flax seeds.

Directions:

1. In a bowl, mix all of the ingredients.
2. Store: Keep in an airtight container in a cold, dry location.

Nutritional value (per serving):

Mixed nuts and seeds include a wealth of nutrients. They are rich in protein, fiber, healthy fats, vitamins, and minerals.

Health benefits:

- **Protein Powerhouse:** Aids in tissue building and repair.
- **Fiber-rich:** Promotes digestion and satiety.
- **Healthy Fats:** Support heart health and brain function.
- **Vitamin and Mineral-rich:** Essential for overall health.
- **Antioxidant-rich:** Protects cells from damage.

Portions per Day: A 1/4-cup portion can be a filling snack.

Note: These nutritional values are approximate and may differ based on the brand and serving size. Always check the nutritional information on the product label.

CHAPTER FIVE
DESSERT
RECIPES

Desserts are a delightful way to end a meal, but they don't have to be overly indulgent to be satisfying. These dessert recipes are designed to be lower in calories while still offering the sweetness and enjoyment you crave. Whether you're in the mood for a creamy treat, a fruity bite, or something chocolate, these desserts will allow you to satisfy your sweet tooth without straying from your 1200-calorie plan. Indulge guilt-free and discover how you can create delicious desserts that fit perfectly into a healthy lifestyle.

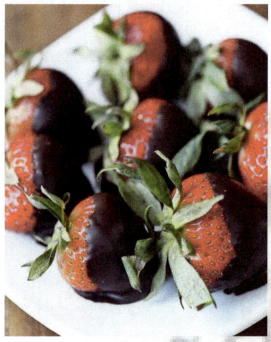

Dark chocolate-dipped strawberries.

Prep Time: 15 minutes

Set Time: 30 minutes

Ingredients:

- 12 big hulled and dried strawberries,
- 8 ounces chopped high-quality dark chocolate, and
- Optional sprinkles, almonds, or coconut flakes for decorating.

Directions:

1. Prepare Strawberries: Wash and thoroughly dry the strawberries.
2. Melt Chocolate: In a double boiler or microwave-safe basin, melt the dark chocolate in short bursts, stirring in between each one.
3. Dip Strawberries: Dip each strawberry in the melted chocolate, covering fully.
4. Optional Toppings: Sprinkle with your favorite toppings just after dipping.
5. Set: Transfer the coated strawberries to a baking sheet lined with wax paper.
6. Chill: Refrigerate for 30 minutes, or until the chocolate has set.

Nutritional value (per serving):

The nutritional content of dark chocolate-dipped strawberries varies according to the type of chocolate and the size of the strawberries. However, here's an overall estimate:

Calories: 80-120, Protein: 1-2g, Fat: 5-8g, Carbs: 10-15g, Sugar: 6-10g, Fiber: 1-2g

Health benefits:

- **Antioxidants:** Dark chocolate contains antioxidants, which can help protect cells from harm.
- **Heart Health:** Dark chocolate contains flavonoids, which can help lower blood pressure and cholesterol levels.
- **Mood Booster:** Dark chocolate can boost mood and reduce stress.
- **Nutrient-Dense:** Strawberries are rich in vitamin C, fiber, and antioxidants.

Portions per Day: A portion of 2–3 dark chocolate-dipped strawberries might be a tasty snack.

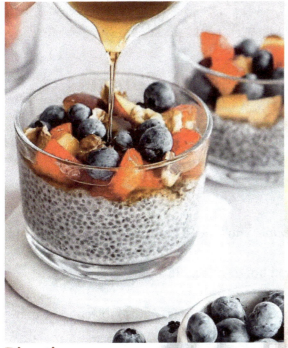

Chia pudding with almond milk

Preparation Time: 5 minutes

Cooking Time: 2 hours or overnight

Ingredients:

- 1/4 cup chia seeds, 1 cup unsweetened almond milk,
- 1 teaspoon maple syrup or honey (optional),
- 1/4 teaspoon vanilla extract.
- Toppings include fresh fruit, almonds, seeds, and coconut flakes.

Directions:

1. Combine Ingredients: In a jar or dish, mix together chia seeds, almond milk, maple syrup, and vanilla essence.
2. Mix Well: Stir until well blended.
3. Chill: Cover and refrigerate for at least 2 hours or overnight.
4. Serve: Chill and top with your favorite fruit, nuts, or seeds.

Nutritional value (per serving):

Calories: 150-200, Protein: 5-8 grams, Fat: 5-10 grams, Carbohydrates: 15-20 grams, Fiber: 5-8 grams, Omega-3 Fatty Acids: Rich in plant-based omega-3s.

Health benefits:

- Fiber promotes digestion and fullness.
- Omega-3 fatty acids support heart health and cognitive function.
- Plant-based protein aids in tissue repair.
- Calcium and Vitamin D are essential for healthy bones and teeth.
- Can be customized with different toppings to suit your preferences.

Portions per Day: One-cup servings can be a filling breakfast or snack.

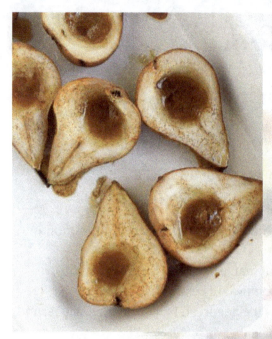

Baked Pears with Cinnamon

Preparation Time: 10 minutes

Cooking Time: 30-40 minutes.

Ingredients:

- For this recipe, you'll need 2 peeled, cored, and halved pears,
- 1 tablespoon honey or maple syrup,
- 1/2 teaspoon ground cinnamon,
- 1/4 teaspoon ground nutmeg, and 1 tablespoon water.

Directions:

1. Preheat your oven to 375°F (190°C).
2. Prepare Pears: Arrange pear halves in a baking dish.
3. Add Sweetener and Spices: Drizzle with honey or maple syrup, then sprinkle with cinnamon and nutmeg.
4. Add Water: Place 1 tablespoon of water in the baking dish.
5. Bake: Cook for 30–40 minutes, or until the pears are soft.
6. Serve: Warm or cold.

Nutritional value (per serving): Calories: 100-150, Fiber: 4-6 grams, Vitamin C: A healthy source, Potassium: important for heart health and blood pressure management.

Health benefits:

- **Rich in fiber:** promotes digestion and keeps you full.
- **Antioxidant powerhouse:** protects cells from damage.
- **Heart-healthy:** lowers cholesterol and reduces risk of heart disease.
- **Hydrating:** high water content keeps you hydrated.
- **Natural sweetener:** a healthier alternative to sugary desserts.

Portions per Day: One cooked pear can serve as a delicious dessert or snack.

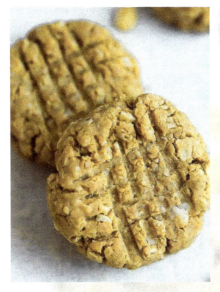

Protein-Rich Peanut Butter Cookies

Prep Time: 15 minutes

Cooking Time: 10-12 minutes

Ingredients:

- 1 cup natural, creamy peanut butter,
- 1/2 cup brown sugar,
- 1 big egg, 1 teaspoon vanilla extract,
- 1/2 teaspoon baking soda,
- 1/4 teaspoon salt,
- 1 cup rolled oats, and
- 1/4 cup chocolate chips (optional).

Directions:

1. Preheat your oven to 350°F (175°C).
2. Combine wet ingredients: In a large mixing basin, combine the peanut butter, brown sugar, egg, and vanilla essence. Beat until thoroughly blended.
3. Add Dry Ingredients: Mix in the baking soda, salt, oats, and chocolate chips (if using).
4. Form Cookies: Drop rounded table spoonfuls onto a baking sheet lined with parchment paper.
5. Bake: Cook for 10 to 12 minutes, or until golden brown.
6. Cool: Allow a few minutes to cool on the baking sheet before transferring to a wire rack to finish cooling.

Nutritional value (per serving): The nutritional value will vary according to the individual ingredients utilized. Peanut butter cookies are, on the whole, high in protein, healthy fats, and fiber.

Health benefits:

- **Protein-Packed:** Aids in tissue building and repair.
- **Healthy Fats:** Promotes heart health and brain function.
- **Fiber-Rich:** Promotes digestion and satiety.
- **Energy Boosting:** Provides long-lasting energy.

Portions per Day: One or two cookies might be a sufficient snack.

BONUS
RECIPES

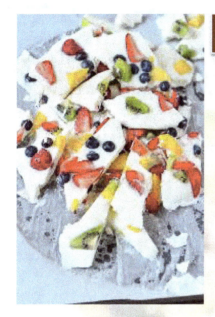

Frozen Yogurt Bark and Fruit

Preparation Time: 10 minutes.

Freezing Time: 2-3 hours.

Ingredients:

- Two cups of Greek yogurt.
- Combine 1/4 cup honey or maple syrup,
- 1 teaspoon vanilla extract,
- 1 cup mixed berries (strawberries, blueberries, raspberries),
- 1/4 cup chopped nuts (almonds, walnuts, pecans), and
- 1/4 cup chocolate chips.

Directions:

1. Line a baking sheet with parchment paper.
2. Combine yogurt ingredients: In a dish, mix together Greek yogurt, honey, and vanilla essence.
3. Spread Yogurt: Spread the yogurt mixture evenly on the prepared baking sheet.
4. Toppings: Garnish with berries, almonds, and chocolate chips.
5. Freeze for 2-3 hours, or until solid.
6. Break into Pieces: Cut the frozen yogurt bark into chunks and serve.

Nutritional value (per serving):

The nutritional value will vary according to the individual ingredients utilized. However, frozen yogurt bark contains protein, calcium, and probiotics.

Health benefits:

- **Protein-Packed:** Promotes tissue repair and gut health.
- **Probiotics:** Promote gut health.
- **Calcium-rich:** Strengthens bones and teeth.
- **Antioxidant-Packed:** Protects cells from damage.
- **Refreshing and Healthy:** A tasty and healthful treat.

Portions per Day: A half-cup portion can be a filling snack.

Note: These nutritional values are approximate and may differ based on the brand and serving size. Always check the nutritional information on the product label.

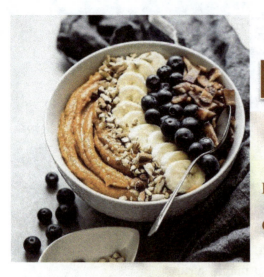

Sweet Potato Breakfast Bowl.

Preparation Time: 10 minutes

Cooking Time: 20-25 minutes

Ingredients:

- 1 big sweet potato (peeled and diced),
- 1/2 cup Greek yogurt, 1/4 cup mixed berries,
- 1 tablespoon chia seeds, and
- 1 teaspoon honey or maple syrup (optional).

Directions:

1. Preheat your oven to 400°F (200°C).
2. Toss sweet potato cubes with olive oil and salt.
3. Roast Sweet Potato: Place sweet potato cubes on a baking sheet and roast for 20 to 25 minutes, or until cooked.
4. Prepare dish: In a mixing dish, add Greek yogurt, mixed berries, and chia seeds.
5. Add Sweet Potato: Serve with roasted sweet potato cubes.
6. Optional: Drizzle with honey or maple syrup.

Nutritional value (per serving): Calories: 300-400, Protein: 15-20 g, Carbohydrates: 40-50 g, Fiber: 6-8 g, Vitamin A: Good source of vitamin A.

Health benefits:

- Fiber promotes digestion and fullness.
- High in Vitamin A, which supports eye health and immunological function.
- Potassium, which helps control blood pressure.
- Protein, which promotes muscle growth and repair.

Portions per Day: A single bowl might be a filling breakfast or a light lunch.

Note: These nutritional values are approximate and may differ based on the brand and serving size. Always check the nutritional information on the product label.

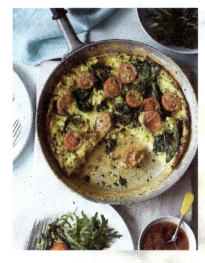

Tomato and Spinach Omelet

Prep Time: 10 minutes

Cooking Time: 5-7 minutes

Ingredients:

- To prepare, combine 2 big eggs,
- 1/4 cup chopped fresh spinach,
- 1/2 small diced tomato,
- 1 tablespoon butter or olive oil, salt, and pepper to taste.
- Optional: feta cheese, shredded cheddar cheese, or any chosen cheese.

Directions:

1. Prepare the vegetables: chop the spinach and tomato into tiny pieces.
2. Whisk the Eggs: In a bowl, beat the eggs until smooth.
3. Cook the Omelette: Heat butter or olive oil in a non-stick pan over medium heat. Pour the whisked eggs into the pan and allow them to set slightly.
4. Add the Fillings: Spread the spinach and tomato over the half-set egg.
5. Flip the Omelette: When the eggs are almost done, use a spatula to flip one side of the omelet over the other, securing the contents within.
6. Optional: Sprinkle your choice of cheese over the folded omelette.
7. Cook Until Done: Continue cooking until the eggs are completely set and the cheese, if used, has melted.
8. Serve: Serve hot with your preferred side dishes, such as bread, fruit, or a salad.

Approximate Nutritional Value: Calories: 150-200 * Protein: 12-15 grams * Fat: 5-8 grams * Carbohydrates: 2-5 grams.

Health benefits:

- **Protein-Packed:** Contains important amino acids for muscle repair and growth.
- **Nutrient-Dense:** Includes vitamins, minerals, and antioxidants from spinach and tomatoes.
- **Low-Calorie:** A light and healthy lunch option.
- **Customizable:** Can be tailored to meet your dietary requirements and tastes.

Portions per Day: A single omelette may be a filling breakfast or a light lunch.

Enjoy this tasty and healthful omelet!

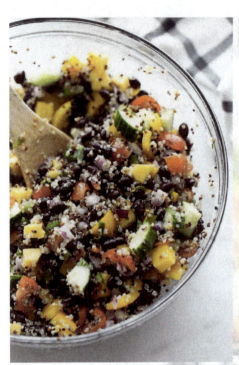

Quinoa and Black Bean Bowl

Prep Time: 15 minutes
Cooking time: 20 to 25 minutes.

Ingredients:

- 1 cup washed quinoa, 1 can (15 oz) rinsed and drained black beans, 1 diced bell pepper, and
- 1/2 cup corn kernels.
- 1/4 cup diced red onion
- 1/4 cup of fresh cilantro, chopped

For the dressing:

- 2 tablespoons of lime juice.
- 1 tablespoon of olive oil.
- 1 teaspoon of cumin.
- 1/2 teaspoon of chili powder.
- Add salt and pepper to taste.

Directions:

1. Cook the Quinoa: Rinse the quinoa and cook according to package instructions.
2. Prepare the vegetables. Chop the bell pepper and red onion.
3. Make the dressing: In a small bowl, whisk together lime juice, olive oil, cumin, chili powder, salt, and pepper.
4. Combine Ingredients: In a large bowl, mix the cooked quinoa, black beans, bell pepper, corn, red onion, and cilantro.
5. Dress the salad: Toss the salad with the dressing until well coated.
6. Serve immediately or keep in an airtight jar in the refrigerator.

Nutritional Value (approximate): Calories: 300–400, Protein: 15-20 g, Carbohydrates: 40 to 50 grams, Fiber: 8–10 grams.

Health Benefits:

- High protein content promotes muscle development and repair.
- High in fiber: aids digestion and keeps you full.

- Packed with vitamins and minerals: Provides critical elements for good health.
- Calories are low, making it an excellent alternative for weight control.
- Versatile: Serve as a main entrée or side dish.
- This substantial and tasty bowl is an excellent way to get more plant-based protein and fiber into your diet. Enjoy!

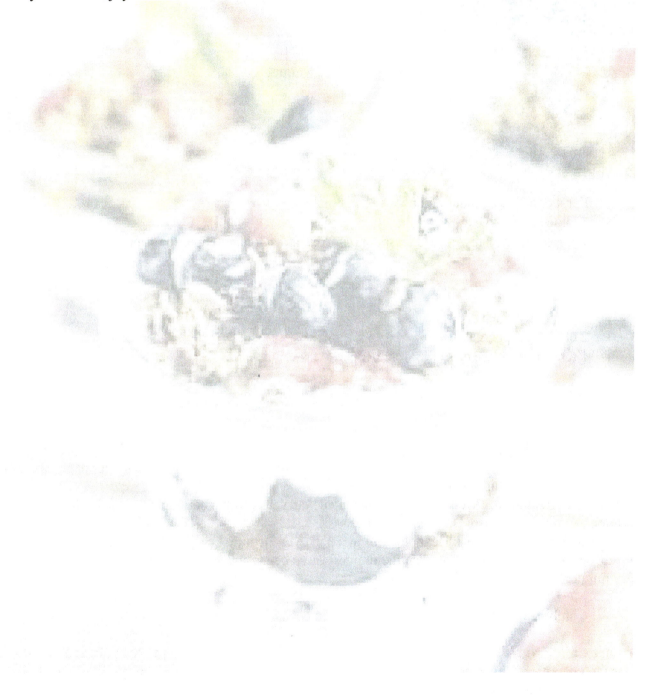

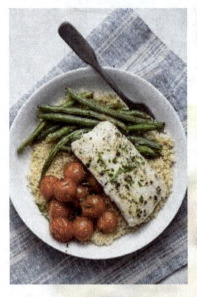

Cod and Garlic Green Beans

Prep Time: 15 minutes

Cooking Time: 20-25 minutes

Ingredients:

For cod:

- For 4 cod fillets (about 6 ounces each), combine
- 1 tablespoon olive oil,
- 1 teaspoon dried thyme, 1/2 teaspoon paprika and salt and pepper to taste.

For green beans:

- 1 pound trimmed green beans,
- 2 cloves chopped garlic,
- 1 tablespoon olive oil, and salt & pepper to taste.

Directions:

1. Preheat your oven to 400°F (200°C).
2. Prepare the fish: To season the fish fillets, combine olive oil, thyme, paprika, salt, and pepper.
3. Roast the Cod: Place the seasoned cod fillets on a baking sheet lined with parchment paper and bake for 15-20 minutes, or until readily flaked with a fork.
4. Cook the green beans: Heat a saucepan of salted water to a boil. Cook the green beans for 3-5 minutes, until tender-crisp. Drain the green beans.
5. To Sauté the Green Beans: Heat olive oil in a pan over medium heat. Add the minced garlic and heat for 30 seconds, or until fragrant. Add the drained green beans and season with salt and pepper. Sauté for 2-3 minutes, or until cooked through.

Serve: Combine the roasted cod and garlicky green beans.

Approximate Nutritional Value: The nutritional value will vary according to the ingredients and portion quantities. However, this meal has a considerable amount of protein, omega-3 fatty acids, vitamins, and minerals.

Health benefits:

- Cod is low in saturated fat, making it a lean protein source.
- Omega-3 fatty acids are beneficial for heart health and cognitive function.
  Vitamins and Minerals: Green beans include vitamins A, C, and K, as well as dietary fiber that assist digestion.

Portions per Day:

A single dish of fish with green beans may be both filling and nutritious.

Enjoy this simple yet wonderful lunch!

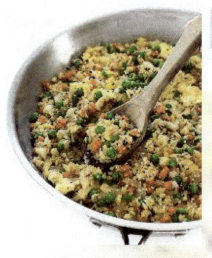

Cauliflower Fried Rice

Prep Time: 15 minutes
Cooking time: 20 to 25 minutes.

Ingredients:

- 1 head of cauliflower riced
- 2 tablespoons of soy sauce.
- 1 tablespoon of oyster sauce.
- 1 teaspoon of sesame oil.
- 2 garlic cloves, minced
- One egg, beaten
- 2 green onions, thinly sliced
- 1/4 cup peas, fresh or frozen
- 1/4 cup shredded carrots.
- Add salt and pepper to taste.

Directions:

1. Cook the cauliflower rice: steam or sauté it until soft and crisp.
2. Prepare the vegetables. Cook the garlic, green onions, peas, and carrots in a pan with a little oil until softened.
3. Scramble the Egg: In a separate pan, cook the eggs.
4. In a large pan, mix together the cooked cauliflower rice, sautéed veggies, scrambled egg, soy sauce, oyster sauce, and sesame oil.
5. Season and serve. Season with salt and pepper to taste. Serve hot.

Nutritional Value (approximate): Calories: 200–300, Protein: 10-15 g, Carbohydrates: 20-30g, Fiber: 5–8 grams

Health Benefits:

- **Low-Carb:** An excellent choice for individuals on a low-carbohydrate diet.
- **High fiber:** content promotes digestion and fullness.
- **Nutrient dense:** high in vitamins, minerals, and antioxidants.
- **Versatile:** Can be adapted with a variety of veggies and protein sources. Portion per day:

This cauliflower fried rice recipe is a tasty and healthier alternative to classic fried rice. Enjoy!

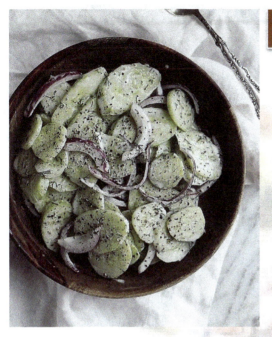

Greek yogurt with cucumber and dill is a refreshing and healthy snack.

Ingredients:

- 1 cup Greek yogurt.
- 1/2 cucumber, peeled, seeded, and chopped
- Add 1 tablespoon chopped fresh dill and 1 tablespoon lemon juice.
- Add salt and pepper to taste.

Directions:

- In a bowl, add Greek yogurt, cucumber, dill, lemon juice, salt, and pepper.
- Mix well. Stir until well blended.
- Chill and Serve: Refrigerate for at least 30 minutes before serving.

Nutritional Value (approximate): Calories: 150–200, Protein: 10-15 g, Fat: 5–8 grams, Carbohydrate content: 10 to 15 grams.

Health Benefits:

- **Protein-Packed:** Contains vital amino acids for muscle repair and development.
  Cucumber has a high water content, which helps you stay hydrated.
  Greek yogurt is probiotic-rich, which promotes digestive health.
- **Low in calories:** A light and pleasant snack.
  Portion per day:

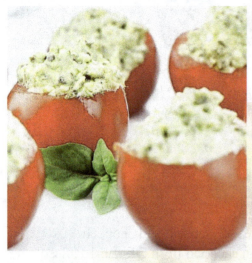

Avocado-stuffed cherry tomatoes

Ingredients:

- To prepare, combine 1 pint cherry tomato,
- 1 ripe avocado,
- 1 tablespoon lime juice,
- 1/4 teaspoon salt,
- 1/4 teaspoon black pepper and chopped fresh cilantro (optional).

Directions:

1. Prepare the tomatoes: Cut a tiny slice off the top of each cherry tomato, then scoop out the seeds.
2. Mash the Avocado: In a small mixing bowl, mash the avocado with a fork until it reaches the required smoothness.
3. Season the Avocado: Combine lime juice, salt, and pepper with the mashed avocado and combine thoroughly.
4. Fill each tomato with the avocado mixture.
5. For garnish: If preferred, sprinkle with fresh cilantro.

Serve immediately.

Approximate Nutritional Value: Each serving has 50–70 calories. Avocado contains healthy fats. Tomatoes and avocados provide vitamins and minerals. Avocado and tomato skins contain fiber.

Health benefits:

Avocados and tomatoes are strong in antioxidants, heart-healthy monounsaturated fats, and high water content. They are also fiber-rich, which aids digestion and satiety.

Portions per Day: A few of these may make a pleasant and nutritious snack.

These avocado-stuffed cherry tomatoes make a tasty and healthy appetizer or snack. They're simple to prepare and ideal for gatherings or potlucks.

Raspberry Coconut Energy Balls.

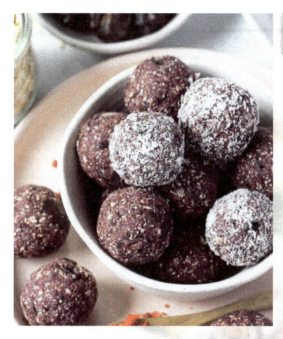

Ingredients:

- 1 cup rolled oats,
- 1/2 cup shredded coconut,
- 1/4 cup chia seeds,
- 1/4 cup honey,
- 1/4 cup peanut butter,
- 1/2 cup fresh or frozen raspberries and 1 teaspoon vanilla extract.

Directions:

1. Mix dry ingredients: In a bowl, mix the rolled oats, shredded coconut, and chia seeds.
2. Combine wet ingredients: In a separate dish, combine the honey, peanut butter, and vanilla essence.
3. Combine wet and dry components: Mix the wet components with the dry ones until thoroughly blended.
4. Gently fold in the raspberries.
5. Form Balls: Shape the mixture into balls about 1 inch in diameter.
6. Chill: Place the energy balls in the refrigerator for at least 30 minutes before serving.

Approximate Nutritional Value:

The nutritional value will vary according to the ingredients and portion quantities. Energy balls, on the other hand, are often high in fiber, protein, and healthy fats.

Health benefits:

- **Energy Boost:** The combination of carbohydrates, protein, and healthy fats provides sustained energy.
- **Rich in Fiber:** Fiber aids digestion and promotes satiety.
- **Antioxidant-Packed:** Raspberries are a beneficial source of antioxidants.
- **Plant-Based Protein:** Peanut butter and chia seeds contain plant-based protein.

Portions per Day: 2-3 energy balls can be a filling and nutritious snack.

These energy balls are an excellent method to refuel your body while satisfying your sweet tooth. They're ideal for a quick breakfast, a midday snack, or a pre-workout boost.

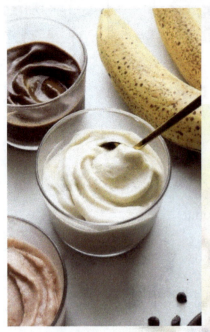

Banana Nice Cream.

Ingredients:

- 2 peeled and frozen bananas,
- 1/4 cup milk (dairy or plant-based),
- 1 tablespoon honey or maple syrup (optional),
- 1/2 teaspoon vanilla extract and toppings such as fresh berries, almonds, chocolate chips, or coconut flakes.

Directions:

1. Freeze Bananas: Peel and slice ripe bananas before freezing them on a baking sheet coated with parchment paper.
2. Blend Ingredients: In a high-speed blender, mix frozen bananas, milk, sweetener, and vanilla extract. Blend until smooth and creamy.
3. Adjust the consistency: If the mixture is too thick, add additional milk. If it's too thin, add some more frozen bananas.
4. Serve: Serve immediately, garnished with your preferred toppings.

Approximate Nutritional Value: The nutritional value will vary according to the ingredients and portion quantities. However, banana lovely cream contains potassium, fiber, and vitamins.

Health benefits:

- Bananas are a natural sweetener with no added sugars.
- They are high in potassium, which helps regulate blood pressure and muscle function.
- They are fiber-rich, which promotes digestion and satiety.
- They are dairy-free, making them a great option for those with allergies or intolerances.
- They are customizable. Can be customized with different toppings to suit your tastes.

Portions per Day:

- A single serving can be a tasty and nutritious dessert or snack.
- This tasty and healthy dessert is a great substitute for regular ice cream. Enjoy!

Creating a Weekly Menu: A Strategic Approach

"UNDERSTANDING YOUR NEEDS"

Before going into meal planning, consider the following factors:

- **Dietary Restrictions:** Are you vegetarian, vegan, gluten-free, or have any other dietary requirements?
- **Time Constraints:** How much time can you devote to meal preparation each week?
- **Taste Preferences:** What kinds of cuisines do you like?
- **Budget:** How much do you want to spend on groceries?
- **Fitness Goals:** Are you striving for weight loss, muscle gain, or overall health?

Developing a balanced meal plan

- A well-balanced meal plan should contain items from each food category.
- This is a simple template:
- Protein provides energy and aids in tissue repair.
- Carbohydrates fuel the body and brain.
- Healthy fats are essential for numerous physical functions.
- Fruits and vegetables include vitamins, minerals, and antioxidants.

MEAL PLANNING TIP

1. Begin with a Basic Template: Breakfast: oatmeal, yogurt with fruit, or eggs Lunch: Salads, sandwiches, or leftovers.
Dinner: Protein (chicken, fish, tofu), carbs (rice, pasta, quinoa), and vegetables. **Snacks:** Fruits, almonds, yogurt, or dark chocolate.

2. Consider Your Lifestyle: For busy weekdays, choose quick and simple meals such as stir-fries, soups, or one-pot recipes.

- **Weekends:** Prepare more complex dinners, such as roasted chicken or handmade pizza.

3. Use Meal Prep Techniques: Cook Once, Eat Twice: Double recipes and freeze leftovers for future meals.

- **Prepare ingredients beforehand of time:** Chop vegetables, marinade meats, and measure out ingredients.
- **Assemble Meals Ahead of Time:** Make salads, sandwiches, or breakfast parfaits beforehand.

4. Incorporate Variety:

- **Switch Up Proteins:** Experiment with various meats, fish, tofu, or lentils. Experiment with grains such as quinoa, brown rice, or farro. Experiment with flavors by including different herbs, spices, and sauces.

SAMPLE WEEKLY MEAL PLAN

Monday:

- **Breakfast:** oatmeal with fruit and almonds.
- **Lunch:** Leftover roasted chicken salad.
- **Dinner:** Grilled salmon and roasted veggies.

Tuesday.

- **Breakfast:** yogurt with honey and granola.
- **Lunch:** lentil soup and whole-grain roll
- **Dinner:** stir-fry with tofu and veggies.

Wednesday:

- **Breakfast:** scrambled eggs on whole grain bread. Lunch: Leftover stir-fry. Dinner: spaghetti with marinara sauce and meatballs.

Thursday:

- **Breakfast:** Smoothie with fruit and yogurt.
- **Lunch:** Tuna salad sandwich on whole wheat bread.
- **Dinner:** Chicken curry with brown rice.

Friday:

- **Breakfast:** avocado toast with a fried egg.
- **Lunch:** Leftover pasta.
- **Dinner:** pizza night.

Weekend plans include brunch (pancakes or waffles with fruit) and supper out on Saturday and Sunday. Roast chicken, potatoes, and veggies

ADDITIONAL TIPS

- Involve your family in meal planning.
- Be flexible and experiment with new recipes and ingredients.
- Set aside time on weekends to prep meals for the week.
- Many applications can help you plan meals, manage your nutrition, and create grocery lists.

By following these guidelines and developing a well-balanced meal plan, you may make healthy eating a permanent part of your lifestyle.

Prepping for Success: A Guide to Meal Planning and Preparation

MEAL PLANNING: THE FOUNDATION

Meal planning is the foundation for successful meal preparation. It enables you to:

- **Save Time**: Planning your meals ahead of time allows you to spend less time determining what to cook.
- **Reduce Food Waste:** Planning your meals allows you to purchase only what you need.
- **Eat Healthier:** A well-planned meal plan ensures that you are eating a balanced diet.
- **Save Money**: Planning your meals allows you to prevent impulse grocery store purchases.

TIPS FOR SUCCESSFUL MEAL PLANNING:

1. **Assess Your Lifestyle:** Consider your job schedule, family responsibilities, and dietary limitations.
2. **Choose dishes:** Choose meals that suit your taste preferences and nutritional requirements.
3. **Create a Weekly Meal Plan:** Outline your meals for the week, including breakfast, lunch, supper, and snacks.
4. **Make a Grocery List:** Utilize your meal plan to build a complete grocery list.
5. **Batch Cook:** To save time, cook big quantities of specific components or recipes at once.

PREP TECHNIQUES: MAXIMIZING YOUR TIME

1. **Wash and chop produce:** Prepare fruits and vegetables in advance and store them in sealed containers.
2. **Marinate Proteins:** Before cooking, marinate meat, poultry, or tofu to tenderize and flavor it.
3. **Cook Grains:** Prepare grains such as rice, quinoa, or pasta in large amounts and keep in the refrigerator or freezer.
4. **Prepare sauces and dressings:** Make sauces and dressings ahead of time and store in jars or bottles.
5. **Assemble Meals:** Prepare meals in sections, such as salad bowls or sandwich components, and refrigerate them.

ADJUSTING RECIPES FOR YOUR TASTE

Once you've established a strong meal plan and preparation routine, you may tailor recipes to your preferences. Here are a few tips:

1. **Spice It Up: Use** additional herbs, spices, or spicy sauce in your food.
2. **Go Low-Calorie:** Choose low-fat options such as Greek yogurt or skim milk.
3. **Increase Protein:** Add additional protein-rich meals like chicken, tofu, or lentils.

4. Lower Carbs: Choose low-carb options such as cauliflower rice or zucchini noodles.
5. Experiment with flavors. Try other cuisines or culinary methods.

HANDLING PLATEAUS: OVERCOMING OBSTACLES IN YOUR FITNESS JOURNEY

Plateaus are a typical issue in fitness. They arise when development appears to stagnate despite sustained effort. Here are some ideas for overcoming plateaus and continuing your fitness quest.

1. Reassess Your Routine:

- To shock your muscles, vary your workouts by introducing new exercises or changing the sequence of your regimen.
- Change the intensity: Increase the weight, resistance, or pace of your exercises.
- Adjust Your Workout Structure: Experiment with varied rep ranges, sets, and rest times.

2. Prioritize Nutrition:

- **Track Your Consumption:** Keep track of your calorie and macronutrient consumption using a food diary or an app.
- **Adjust Your Diet:** If you aren't seeing results, try raising or lowering your calorie consumption.
- **Optimize Your Macronutrient Ratio:** Make sure you're getting the correct mix of protein, carbs, and fat.

3. Managing Stress:

- **Practice Mindfulness:** Techniques such as meditation and yoga can help decrease stress and enhance general wellbeing.
- **Prioritize Sleep:** Proper sleep is essential for recuperation and hormone control.
- **Manage Stressors:** Determine and handle the causes of stress in your life.

4. Be patient and persistent:

- Break down larger goals into smaller, achievable steps.
- Celebrate small wins and acknowledge progress.
- Stay motivated by listening to music, watching fitness videos, or joining a community.

5. Seek professional guidance:

- **Ask a fitness trainer:** A certified trainer can assist you in developing a specific training plan as well as providing coaching on form and technique.

- **Ask a registered dietician:** A nutritionist may assist you in developing a dietary plan that aligns with your fitness objectives.
- Remember that plateaus are a natural part of the fitness process. By applying these tactics, you may overcome difficulties and continue to grow toward your goals.
- Would you like to explore further into a certain component of fitness, such as strength training, cardio, or nutrition? Or maybe you'd want to talk about how to stay motivated to exercise over the long haul.

CELEBRATING MILESTONES: THE KEY TO LONG-TERM FITNESS SUCCESS

Celebrating milestones is an effective way to stay motivated and achieve long-term fitness achievements. Recognizing your accomplishments may raise your self-esteem, increase your motivation, and help you stick to your fitness objectives.

Tips for Celebrating Fitness Milestones:

- **Set clear goals:** Establish precise, measurable, attainable, relevant, and time-bound (SMART) fitness objectives. This will allow you to monitor your progress and identify milestones.
- **Track Your Progress:** Use a fitness notebook, app, or wearable device to track your workouts, nutrition, and other pertinent data. This will allow you to better visualize your progress and identify areas for improvement.
- **Reward Yourself:** When you achieve a goal, treat yourself to something you love, such as new exercise attire, a massage, or a nutritious snack.
- **Share Your Success:** Inform your friends, family, and the internet community about your accomplishments. Sharing your accomplishments may keep you motivated and encourage others.
- **Reflect on Your Journey:** Spend some time reflecting on how far you've come and the obstacles you've conquered. This might help you recognize your accomplishments and remain motivated for future ambitions.

Stay Motivated: Tips and Tricks

- **Find Your Why:** Identify your motivations for achieving your fitness objectives. Having a strong "why" can help you stay motivated even when things are difficult.
- **Make Fitness Fun:** Choose activities that you like and make you feel good. This will help you stay motivated and incorporate exercise into your daily routine.
- **Set realistic goals:** Establish attainable goals that you can work toward gradually. This will prevent you from feeling overwhelmed and discouraged.
- **Find an exercise buddy:** Having an exercise companion may keep you accountable and motivated.

- **Celebrate Non-Scale Victories:** Concentrate on other indicators of success, such as more energy, better sleep, or improved mood.
- **Do Not Be Afraid to Take Breaks: It** is OK to break from your usual routine. A little break might help you recover and return stronger.
- **Visualize Your Success:** Imagine yourself attaining your fitness objectives. This might help you maintain motivation and attention.

By celebrating your accomplishments and staying motivated, you may reach your fitness objectives and live a healthier, happier lifestyle.

60-Day Meal Plan

Week 1-2:

- Day 1-3:

    - **Breakfast**: Greek Yogurt Parfait with Berries
    - **Lunch**: Grilled Chicken Salad with Lemon Dressing
    - **Dinner**: Baked Salmon with Asparagus
    - **Snack**: Veggie Sticks with Hummus

- Day 4-6:

    - **Breakfast**: Banana-Oat Pancakes
    - **Lunch**: Zucchini Noodles with Marinara Sauce
    - **Dinner**: Grilled Shrimp Tacos with Salsa
    - **Snack**: Veggie Sticks with Hummus

- Day 7:

    - **Breakfast**: Spinach and Mushroom Egg Muffins
    - **Lunch**: Turkey and Avocado Sandwich on Whole Grain
    - **Dinner**: Chicken Stir-Fry with Brown Rice
    - **Snack**: Veggie Sticks with Hummus

Week 3-4:

- Day 8-10:

    - **Breakfast**: Avocado Toast with a Poached Egg
    - **Lunch**: Grilled Chicken Salad with Lemon Dressing
    - **Dinner**: Stuffed Bell Peppers with Quinoa
    - **Snack**: Veggie Sticks with Hummus

- Day 11-13:

    - **Breakfast**: Greek Yogurt Parfait with Berries
    - **Lunch**: Zucchini Noodles with Marinara Sauce
    - **Dinner**: Grilled Shrimp Tacos with Salsa
    - **Snack**: Veggie Sticks with Hummus

- **Day 14**:
    - **Breakfast**: Banana-Oat Pancakes
    - **Lunch**: Turkey and Avocado Sandwich on Whole Grain
    - **Dinner**: Chicken Stir-Fry with Brown Rice
    - **Snack**: Veggie Sticks with Hummus

Week 5-6:

- **Day 15-17**:
    - **Breakfast**: Spinach and Mushroom Egg Muffins
    - **Lunch**: Grilled Chicken Salad with Lemon Dressing
    - **Dinner**: Baked Salmon with Asparagus
    - **Snack**: Veggie Sticks with Hummus

- **Day 18-20**:
    - **Breakfast**: Avocado Toast with a Poached Egg
    - **Lunch**: Zucchini Noodles with Marinara Sauce
    - **Dinner**: Stuffed Bell Peppers with Quinoa
    - **Snack**: Veggie Sticks with Hummus

- **Day 21**:
    - **Breakfast**: Greek Yogurt Parfait with Berries
    - **Lunch**: Turkey and Avocado Sandwich on Whole Grain
    - **Dinner**: Grilled Shrimp Tacos with Salsa
    - **Snack**: Veggie Sticks with Hummus

Week 7-8:

- **Day 22-24**:
    - **Breakfast**: Banana-Oat Pancakes
    - **Lunch**: Grilled Chicken Salad with Lemon Dressing
    - **Dinner**: Chicken Stir-Fry with Brown Rice
    - **Snack**: Veggie Sticks with Hummus

- **Day 25-27:**
    - **Breakfast**: Spinach and Mushroom Egg Muffins
    - **Lunch**: Zucchini Noodles with Marinara Sauce
    - **Dinner**: Baked Salmon with Asparagus
    - **Snack**: Veggie Sticks with Hummus

- **Day 28**:
    - **Breakfast**: Avocado Toast with a Poached Egg
    - **Lunch**: Turkey and Avocado Sandwich on Whole Grain
    - **Dinner**: Stuffed Bell Peppers with Quinoa
    - **Snack**: Veggie Sticks with Hummus

Week 9-10:

- **Day 29-31**:
    - **Breakfast**: Greek Yogurt Parfait with Berries
    - **Lunch**: Grilled Chicken Salad with Lemon Dressing
    - **Dinner**: Grilled Shrimp Tacos with Salsa
    - **Snack**: Veggie Sticks with Hummus

- **Day 32-34**:
    - **Breakfast**: Banana-Oat Pancakes
    - **Lunch**: Zucchini Noodles with Marinara Sauce
    - **Dinner**: Chicken Stir-Fry with Brown Rice
    - **Snack**: Veggie Sticks with Hummus

- **Day 35**:
    - **Breakfast**: Spinach and Mushroom Egg Muffins
    - **Lunch**: Turkey and Avocado Sandwich on Whole Grain
    - **Dinner**: Baked Salmon with Asparagus
    - **Snack**: Veggie Sticks with Hummus

DEAR VALUED CUSTOMER,

I hope you are enjoying your freshly acquired book!
I am glad that you chose to invest in my

Product and I appreciate you for that.

I recognize that your time is precious, and I am grateful for any further time you may be able to take to offer an honest evaluation. I feel that customer input is vital, and your opinions will help me produce an even better product in the future.

It would be very appreciated if you could take a few minutes to provide an honest review of this book. I genuinely respect your views and ideas and would be glad to get your suggestions on how I might improve.

I appreciate your devotion to my product, and I thank you for taking the time to offer an honest review.

Best Regard

JEFFREY M. JONES

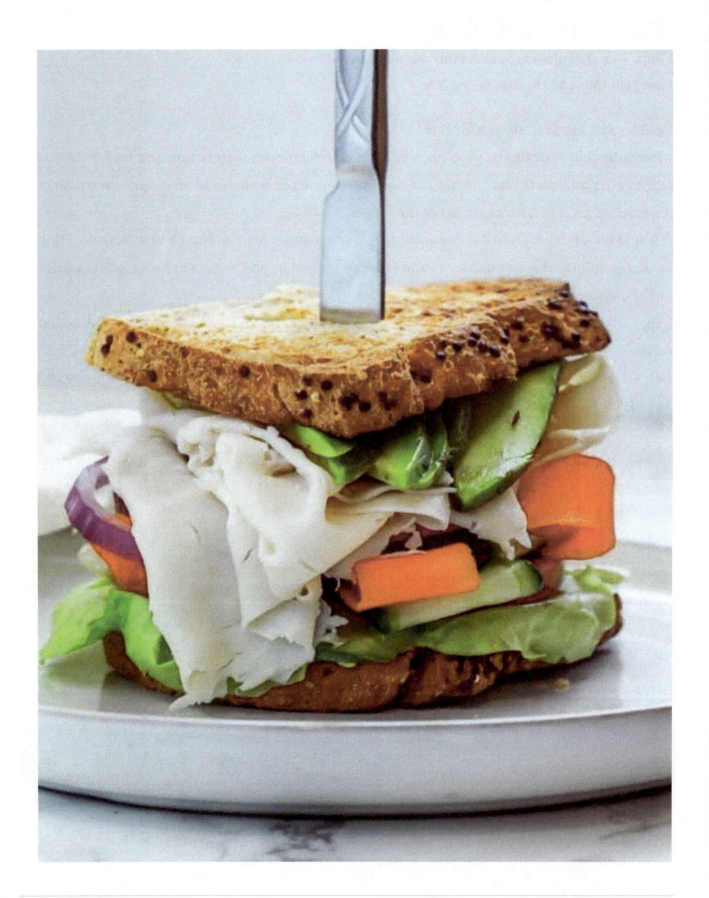

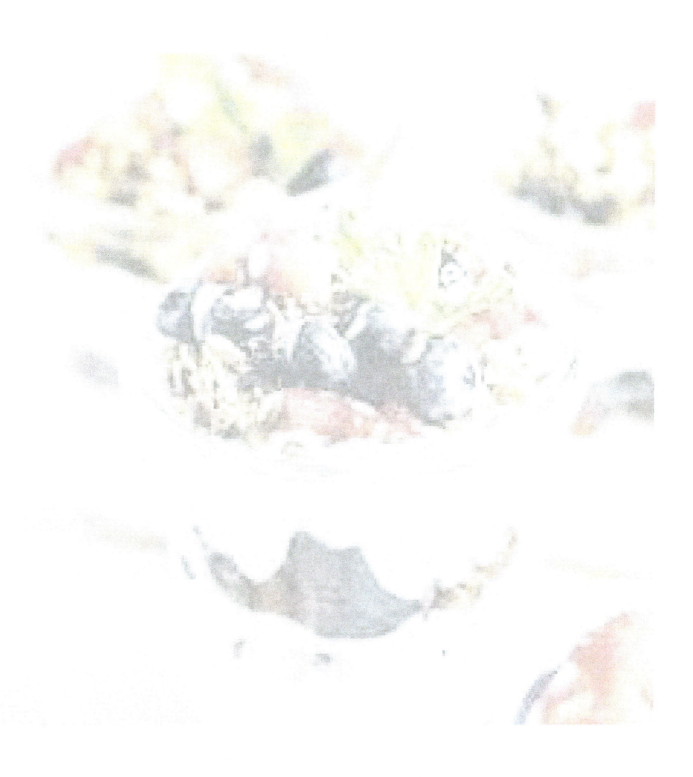

1 | JEFFREY M. JONES COOKBOOK